Health has...

Alf Birken

The role of a physician is usually to diagnose and treat disease but not prevent that disease. Dr. Birken has left that concept behind. Contrary to what most physicians convey to their patients, Dr. Birken introduces the concepts of a healthy life program whereby every day we wake up we experience health and wellness and a better quality of life.
Dr. Neal Rouzier

For the patients who read this book, I know you will find renewed hope that Dr. Birken possesses the key remedy for those symptoms like fatigue, insomnia, weight gain, brain fog, decreased sex drive, and mood swings. His path is not one of antidepressants, sleeping pills, and synthetic hormones.
Dr. Gary Donovitz

Dr. Birken effectively lays out clinical and research based conclusions using real patient data in regards to bioidentical hormone replacement. He pulls no punches as to why Big Pharma does not want patients and physicians to know the truth about their health and what bioidentical hormone replacement can do for the entire population.
Dr. Jasper Lovoi III, Pharm.D.

THE BIO-IDENTICAL WAY: PATIENT PROFILES IN NATURAL HORMONE OPTIMIZATION

THE BIO-IDENTICAL WAY: PATIENT PROFILES IN NATURAL HORMONE OPTIMIZATION

Randy A. Birken M.D.

© 2017 Randy A. Birken M.D.
All rights reserved.

ISBN-13: 9781546457770
ISBN-10: 1546457771

Contents

Foreword

Writing a book to educate and entertain patients is a difficult and formidable task for a physician. However, I am both a physician as well as a patient and therefore understand the thought processes and desires of both. And, therefore, I write this foreword for Dr. Birken from the perspective of a physician as well as a happy, healthy, content, and optimized patient. As Dr. Birken has mentioned throughout his book, he has referenced my book where I discussed medical literature and science but to the detriment of using too much science and not enough case examples. Dr. Birken has fixed this by using his clinical experience and expertise to better educate us and the patient as to the signs and symptoms that various patients will encounter and the benefits and improvements that he and I have witnessed after many years of prescribing BHRT. His use of clinical vignettes drives home the importance of his treatments. Recently I spoke with him about his goal and desire for the book as I was not sure if it was to enlighten physicians or teach and show patients what they are missing. He stated, "My goal is to enlighten patients regarding the clinical approaches for BHRT through, hopefully, engaging narratives; all stories are interspersed with scientific facts that you have taught me." Congratulations, Dr. Birken, as you have done such a fine job of that.

My obsession with demonstrating what the medical literature shows does not bode well in explaining to a reader or a patient how or why they benefit from BHRT. Dr. Birken, however, does a superb job of presenting so many of the scenarios that reinforce the need for BHRT. He does not leave out any scenario where men and women benefit from optimization of hormones. He writes from a patient's perspective and details exactly what patients want to read and experience as opposed to the scientific, boring details that I addressed in my book. For everything that I did wrong, Dr. Birken has done right in speaking from a patient's perspective, and then we follow him through his thought process in helping patients feel and function better. Only with years of training and experience would a physician be able to do so. With Dr. Birken's research and background, years of clinical experience, and a clear desire to help patients outside of the standard paradigm of medicine, Dr. Birken has put together a book that all patients and physicians should embrace. The key to understanding why we do what we do is through the medical literature that demonstrates optimizing hormone levels, not just normalizing, is where patients benefit the most. This concept is not well understood or accepted by most physicians as we simply don't receive this education in our usual training.

Dr. Birken has understood optimal hormone replacement, health and wellness for years and has attended all of the HRT seminars that I teach on optimal health and preventive medicine. Dr. Birken summarizes for us all his research to educate us how to improve and maintain our health and well-being. He even uses himself as a case example of an aging physician, experiencing all the symptoms and ailments of life and how he found solutions for himself. In each chapter, he explains his thought process for each patient. His intent is to introduce us to all the health and wellness benefits of BHRT, diet, exercise, lifestyle change, stress reduction, with focus on mind, body, and soul. I appreciate his intent of convincing the reader to do what all physicians do on a daily basis, which is the very reason we became physicians, and that is to help someone. Dr. Birken derives tremendous satisfaction by simply helping all the people he can. I'm sure that Dr. Birken's main intent of this book is to help the reader understand how to help themselves. The trials and tribulation of practicing medicine are not pleasant and most physicians are unfortunately not happy. Dr. Birken, like many of us who practice BHRT, is thrilled to help patients and we can see the elation in his writing.

This type of practice that we now embrace makes medicine fun again when we truly help people feel better. We have both discovered that helping patients provides us with a sense of accomplishment in life. Dr. Birken so eloquently describes the gratitude that patients have for him and his treatments. This has transformed Dr. Birken into a physician and human being who wants to change lives in a positive manner.

The role of a physician is usually to diagnose and treat disease but not prevent that disease. Dr. Birken has left that concept behind. Contrary to what most physicians convey to their patients, Dr. Birken introduces the concepts of a healthy life program whereby every day we wake up we experience health and wellness and a better quality of life. What a concept, but a concept that all physicians should embrace but many don't. Dr. Birken focuses on every aspect of health, wellness, stress, diet, exercise, BHRT, and how to be the happiest and best person we can be.

More importantly, patients and physicians will come to understand that patients no longer want to go to physicians only to be treated for a disease or illness. Patients now demand that physicians partner with them to prevent disease and illness but also improve quality of life. Dr. Birken teaches us how to prevent disease and illness and at the same time make us feel and function at our optimum. Perhaps an alternative title should have been "Age Healthier, Live Happier, and Enjoy Life to the Utmost" as that is what he conveys in this book. Thank you, Dr. Birken, for taking us down this path of focusing on the patient and not what we were taught conventionally.

Neal Rouzier, M.D.

Introduction

As patients and their physicians meander through the murky waters of healthcare, both are in search of the same thing, "a healthier happy life." In the past, books on healthcare were written either for the patient or for the physician and a dark chasm left each wondering if they were on the same path, with the same goals, and the same desires. I am honored to write the introduction for Dr. Randy Birken's new book *The Bio-Identical Way: Patient Profiles in Natural Hormone Optimization*. I know both patients and practitioners will benefit from the stories of his patients as they experience the life-changing benefits of hormone optimization.

As an obstetrician and a gynecologist, Dr. Birken has been involved in the lifecycle of his patients from teenage, to motherhood and then menopause. Their life experiences have become his, their complaints and therapies have been shared between them, and their stories of how he has changed their lives has empowered him to keep being a great and relevant physician.

As a Board Certified Ob/Gyn, Dr. Birken has had the uphill battle of challenging the Board that certifies him as they continue to dish the utilization of bio-identical hormones. He has continued to champion the battle for compounded bio-identical hormones when big pharmaceutical companies have tried to redirect his patients to synthetic hormones with less benefits and more risk.

I consider Dr. Birken an expert in the field of hormone replacement therapy for both men and women. It was because of his knowledge and his passion for patient "healthier aging" that I asked him to serve on the BioTE Medical Advisory Board for the past four years. He has been generous in sharing his experiences and patient success stories and therapies with BioTE Medical, allowing all our practitioners to benefit their patients from his eighteen-plus years of experience.

The path to hormone optimization is a challenging one because our patients' aging processes are unique. Dr. Birken has adopted a philosophy of hormone individualization that ultimately leads to optimization. He understands the benefits of not overmedicating his patients. His knowledge of the literature and best practices allows him to reduce the chance for heart disease, diabetes mellitus, Alzheimer's disease, breast cancer, and osteoporosis in his patients.

For the patients who read this book, I know you will find renewed hope that Dr. Birken possesses the key remedy for those symptoms like fatigue, insomnia, weight gain, brain fog, decreased sex drive, and mood swings. His path is not one of antidepressants, sleeping pills, and synthetic hormones. Just ask the thousands of men and women of the Houston area who's lives he has transformed.

For the physicians who read this book, maybe it's time you rethink your methods of hormone optimization. Dr. Birken offers you a path with a therapy that has been used for eighty years. The benefits are life changing and the side effects are minimal.

Thanks, Randy, for sharing your life changing stories. They serve as reminder of why we all went to medical school. The information presented allows us to feel your passion for healthcare, your experience with hormone optimization, and relate your life-changing moments with your patients to, hopefully, all who read this book and those we know who would benefit from reading it.

Gary Donovitz, M.D.
CEO and Medical Director, BioTE Medical, LLC
President, Institute for Hormonal Balance
Author, *Age Healthier, Live Happier, Avoiding Over-Medication through Natural Hormone Balance*
International Lecturer, Bio-Identical Hormone Replacement Therapy Using Subcutaneous Pellet Therapy

1

The Bio-Identical Way

It was the end of a long Tuesday at the clinic as I sat at my desk, exhausted, and completed the thirty-plus dictations for patients seen that day. For just a moment, I allowed myself to sit back and close my eyes. I had another two full days of clinic before the all-day Friday surgery schedule. Today, all patient visits are noted through electronic medical records, but in 1999, a transcriptionist would listen to my dictations, print them out, bring them to the office manager the next day, and each section pasted to a sheet that would become part of the patient's records. Antiquated compared to today's technical advances, with the use of templates, electronic prescriptions, labs, and radiology reports neatly entered into easily accessible files. I remember when I moved my office, after twenty-nine years at the same location, to one near my home, requiring boxes and boxes of patient paper charts to be reorganized within two rooms. A year later, I converted to electronic medical records, then another year to scan all the paper charts into the new EMR system—no more charts, no more loose papers, lost reports, and the time required by my staff to find the appropriate file - this was tidy and efficient, everything accessed through a laptop or desktop. Why hadn't I done this before the move and saved myself, and my staff, the aggravation of moving and filing paper charts? I opened my eyes and smiled—that's just life.

I had to make hospital rounds on Monday's surgical patients before heading home. Although usually tired, I would force myself to change into workout clothes and go to the gym, my time to de-stress and revitalize my overwhelmed mind. But it wasn't that easy. Sometimes, I took my patients' problems home, disrupting my thoughts and a good night's rest. Perhaps, as a doctor, I took my role as a caregiver too seriously. My gynecology residency was four years of intense, sleep-deprived work, training, at least I thought, that would allow me to provide answers to my all patients' concerns. But, at times, I felt lost, unable to help menopausal and peri-menopausal patients with their problems—symptoms more than just hot flashes and night sweats, but other concerns such as fatigue, poor sleep, weight gain, reduced libido, mental fog, aches and pains, and of course, the frequent complaint about weight gain—basically, a general compromise to overall vitality and sense of well-being. But why? Consistently, I attended medical meetings and took continuing medical education courses, following my medical specialty's updated recommendations and protocols. Why didn't I have answers to these patient concerns? Surely, not everyone was depressed. Why should I prescribe an anxiolytic or antidepressant such as Prozac or Effexor like many of my colleagues? Why give a patient something that may not help and instead increase lethargy, cause weight gain, and possibly compromise libido? Was this just the aging process? Did my patients have unrealistic expectations promoted by the TV ads and storylines from books and movies? Was I being unrealistic in what I could provide? Life changes as you get older, I would reflect, and being tired, gaining weight, lowered libido, and just looking old were part of the process, or so I thought.

Personally, I was beginning to identify with my patients' complaints, obviously as a male. Soon to be fifty, I was experiencing more fatigue and, despite eating healthy, exercising, and taking appropriate supplements, I too was gaining weight and losing muscle mass. Getting old? Yes. Feeling old? Sadly, yes. And I didn't want to accept it. I needed my strength and stamina—two hundred surgeries a year and over thirty office patients three days per week. Most importantly, I wanted to live wholly, to see, to learn, to be enlightened with the world, to experience everything, and not someone who slowly deteriorates, accepting the aging process regretfully. Yet, was there something else? I'm a physician. Shouldn't I know? Why did my patients, as well as myself, slowly become less agile in body and mind?

It wasn't till a few months later that I discovered a means to feel youthful again, more robust, healthier physically and mentally, and to offer this to my patients whom I had pledged to care for as a physician since I graduated from medical school in 1976.

Surprisingly, it wasn't some new medical discovery or an expensive medication created by the pharmaceutical companies, something developed from plants only to be suppressed by the established medical organizations due to pharmaceutical companies' pressures. No magic potions; no hypnotic methodology; no Eastern medicine discipline (although I embrace meditative mind/body practices). Simply, compounds that were identical to our own molecular substances produced in our bodies. Metabolic and reproductive hormones, natural and recognized by our own physiology. A science – but requiring the art of medicine as well—the process of analyzing hormone levels and customizing a bio-identical protocol that is effective and safe. To regain strength, to improve vigor, to enhance metabolism, to stabilize mood.

Medical establishments, such as conventional medical societies and organizations, frown on how I prescribe these bio-identical hormones. Even physicians, once medical students or interns/residents who trained under my tutelage when I was a faculty member, criticize my protocols. Why? Well, we are all influenced by peer pressure or what is considered "standard" protocols—but these powerful pressures are shaped by self-interest groups, organizations that benefit from the manufacture of synthetic hormones. It took years of seeking alternative education, evidenced-based scientific studies untainted by profit-seeking companies, and data supporting the safety, potency, and long-term benefits of bio-identical hormones. Science that clearly validates how these compounds reduce age-related problems and diseases. The proven data was there but continued to be swept under the rug so patients would be prescribed more drugs for hypertension, diabetes, elevated cholesterol, sleep, and mood.

Dr. Neal Rouzier, in his book, *Natural Hormone Replacement for Men and Women: How to Achieve Healthy Aging*, 2nd edition, writes:

> We now see that when hormones are at optimal levels, the body is healthy and in better physical condition. Sleep, diet, and exercise influence our essential levels; however, by themselves, they do not delay the decline. Physical, emotional, and mental deterioration are also a direct reflection of the state of our hormones. Research demonstrates that the only solution to alter this age-associated decline is through hormone supplementation.

Our hormones keep us healthy and when restored to optimal ranges, they keep us energetic and youthful.

Dr. Gary Donovitz, president and founder of BioTE Medical, is another one of my mentors, offering clinical training to physicians. From his book, *Age Healthier, Live Happier: Avoiding Over-Medication through Hormone Balance*, he writes about low testosterone in males:

The symptoms are an easy way to help make the diagnosis. Men feel fatigued (especially after noon), experience insomnia, and have decreased memory, focus, and concentration. They have "presentisms," where they go to work and they are present and accounted for, but their performance is subpar. Workouts are less productive, and in fact they begin losing muscle mass. Sexual performance is decreased. This is most noticeable by a loss of morning erections and loss of erections after ejaculation. Some men even lose their libido. These symptoms have deleterious effects on a man's relationship with his partner. It is by no coincidence that the peak years of divorce correspond to the early year of menopause.

Vividly, I remember the day I took my first course on bio-identical hormones with Dr. Rouzier—no PowerPoint, just the use of an overhead projector, medical studies with statistically significant conclusions regarding the efficacy, safety, and long-term use of bio-identical hormones. I sat in a small class of approximately twenty to thirty physicians, awed by data that had never been presented to me in continuing education courses before, information that was exciting and fresh. Angrily I thought, why wasn't this taught to me before? Again, from Dr. Rouzier's book:

> Peer reviewed journals in every specialty of medicine back me up. I am able to show cardiologists how testosterone, estrogen, and thyroid are good for the heart. I am able to show internists that thyroid insufficiencies are not always uncovered by TSH tests, and how thyroid may even help a "healthy" patient. To the doctors looking down their noses at natural hormones, I ask you to read your own journals for the information I extol. The justification is present in our medical journals and literature. The data for natural hormones and *against* synthetic hormones is scientific, peer reviewed evidence based in the medical literature.

Should I malign the pharmaceutical industry? Yes, they spend a huge amount of money on research and development, but they are for profit as well as a powerful political force. Another quote from Dr. Donovitz's book regarding the pharmaceutical companies for profit goals:

> Dr. Arnold Relman, Professor Emeritus of Medicine and Social Medicine at *Harvard Medical School*, and past editor of *The New England Journal of Medicine*, reported that Big Pharma spends one-third of all sales revenue on marketing their products—roughly twice what they spend on research and development.
>
> As a result of this drive to maintain sales, there is now, in the words of the World Health Organization (WHO), "an inherent conflict of interest between the legitimate business goals of manufacturers and the social, medical, and economic needs of providers and the public to select and use drugs in the most rational way."

In addition, the pharmaceutical companies spend a significant amount of money to undermine the compounding pharmacies, Independent pharmacists who customized medications as well as bio-identical hormones. In the past, pharmacists made, or compounded, formulations as stipulated by physicians. However, as medications became mass-produced, pharmacists became dispensers for the drug companies' "one-size-fits-all" dosages. Professional Compounders of

America, or PCCA, is an independent compounding pharmacy's resource for training and support to pharmacists. From their website:

> Pharmacy compounding is the art and science of preparing personalized medications for patients. Compounded medications are made based on a practitioner's prescription in which individual ingredients are mixed together in the exact strength and dosage form required by the patient. This method allows the compounding pharmacist to work with the patient and the prescriber to customize a medication to meet the patient's specific needs.

Some physicians feel that they can only prescribe a FDA-approved drug and big pharma exploits this fear to intimidate clinicians. But this "FDA" concept is a fallacy. From PCCA:

> The FDA approval process is intended for mass-produced drugs made by manufacturers. Because compounded medications are personalized for individual patients, the federal government has approved the use of compounded medications for those individuals who have received a prescription for that specific compounded medication.

After all my accredited courses, exams, and hours spent on studying research about bio-identical hormones, how was I to take this new information, this new approach, these new concepts and formulate appropriately compounded natural hormone protocols? How was I to bypass the pharmaceutical companies' influence on prescribing? How could I use this new knowledge—unconventional and alternative—and help my patients restore their vitality? At first, I was overwhelmed. But, I took hold of my concerns and realized there was only one simple approach—by talking with my patients, developing customized hormone compounds, and applying it to different clinical situations. It would take months of "practicing" medicine, reviewing labs, speaking with compounding pharmacists, and meeting again with my patients, to understand the subtleties of this medical approach. But the profuse thanks from patients, those who now experienced more energy, better sleep, weight loss, mood enhancement, improved libido, and overall increase in well-being, was the reward for my efforts... and for me, personally, regaining my strength and stamina, motivation and focus...my old self through bio-identical hormone optimization.

Presented here are various clinical scenarios, composites of real patients, clinical vignettes to teach the many aspects of bio-identical hormone optimization through engaging narratives. We begin with my first bio-identical hormone patient—her complaints, frustrations, and fears until her understanding of the benefits, as well as safety, of natural hormone optimization. Then, a classic middle-aged man who begins to experience a loss of testosterone—his symptoms and dramatic response to treatment. Then to a new clinical problem—a perimenopausal woman desperate to move past tough personal problems to start a new life, but now with restored vitality. Then, a rarely undiagnosed problem in the past but now detected more often—a young male with debilitating low testosterone problems. And finally, the most common endocrine problem among premenopausal women usually missed by standard blood tests—insulin resistance, with its symptoms, potential serious consequences, treatment guidelines, and successful outcomes.

While most patients fall in several different categories, these clinical scenarios are used to illustrate the wide spectrum of hormone deficiencies. But more importantly, to enlighten the reader to the many clinical presentations of hormone deficiencies, the medical implications and effects on energy, weight, mood, sleep, libido, aches and pains, and compromise on overall vitality. These clinical vignettes allow me, the physician, to educate those seeking alternatives to conventional therapies and to validate patients who are already taking natural hormones. A journey not only as a doctor but as a personal commitment to myself and my family. Come join me—learn and embrace.

> *It's not how old you are; it's how you are old.*
>
> JULES RENARD

2

Ellie

Hormone replacement therapy may not be a cure for dying but it makes life longer, exciting, and much more fulfilling. Hormone replacement therapy provides vigor and vitality which would otherwise be lost.

DR. NEAL ROUZIER

NATURAL HORMONE REPLACEMENT FOR MEN AND WOMEN: HOW TO ACHIEVE HEALTHY AGING, 2ND EDITION

Every evening, after returning from Dr. Rouzier's first course, I would study and reread the hundreds of printed notes as well as review the medical studies supporting the use of bio-identical instead of synthetic hormones. In the early days, Dr. Rouzier presented data, rather than a specific plan for optimizing hormones. This wasn't his responsibility, but mine, the physician. I was the one who listened to a patient's concerns, interpreted the blood tests, and recommended a specific, customized protocol. I learned the concepts, but now I needed to apply them appropriately, safely, and most importantly, effectively.

I was eager to offer this alternative hormone approach to my first patient but not without some trepidation. First, would my patients want to try this instead of traditional hormones? Since compounded hormones are not covered by conventional insurance, would patients be willing to pay for the benefits? And most importantly, would they improve clinically with bio-identical hormones rather than synthetic? I understood the scientific data Dr. Rouzier taught, but still, as a traditionally trained gynecologist, was I really doing the right thing?

Ellie, a fifty-four-year-old, was well known to me. Obstetrics was part of my practice the first ten years until I shifted my clinical focus to gynecological surgery and uro-gynecology. I helped birth her last child, now nineteen, and had performed a hysterectomy for endometriosis when Ellie was forty-six years old. At fifty-one, she developed the usual menopausal symptoms—hot flashes, night sweats, poor sleep, mental fog, and reduced libido. She struggled with her decision to take hormones.

"Dr. Birken, I'm worried about starting hormones," she said, her face lined with concern. "My grandmother died of some type of cancer. We don't know what kind but I suspect breast cancer." She sighed. "But I'm miserable with these hot flashes and night sweats!"

And she did look miserable. Her usual happy personality was gone and her healthy skin was now ridden with dark circles of sleep deprivation under her eyes, and a significant increase in wrinkles. This was not an unusual observation—many patients went through this transition, a sudden shift from youthfulness to aging. Silently, I noted her eleven pound weight gain in just one year.

"I didn't expect this," she said with a desperate look I never noticed before. "I'm a strong woman," she continued. "Been able to handle those tough teenage years with my kids. My father's dementia. My sister's divorce. My husband's colon cancer. But now, I can't seem to handle anything. I'm nervous, moody, and look terrible." She lowered her eyes and then looked up with a pleading facial expression. "I need help, Dr. Birken."

I nodded. I had my own mixed feelings about hormones. I knew that estrogen had protection on bones and reduced the risk for colorectal cancer. And yes, for most, alleviation of those debilitating hot flashes. But did it really help reduce heart disease? And did it promote breast cancer? I didn't know. But I was sure Ellie needed help. It saddened me to see her usual cheerful and upbeat persona changed so dramatically.

"Ellie," I said calmly and slowly, "Let's try a low-dose estrogen. Maybe for a month and then reevaluate. If you can sleep and feel better during the day, it's worth it."

She nodded slowly. "Okay. Agreed. One month. Yes. Just one month." She smiled. "Thanks."

In those days, every pharmaceutical company "rep" would extoll the benefits of their hormone product over others. They would "push" their tablets, capsules, patches, rings, and creams based on medical studies, sponsored by their drug company, stating why they were better than the others. I didn't approve of their "bribes" to promote their products. Lunches, pens, pads, even golf balls—it didn't feel right. I wanted the best for my patients, not what benefited me, the prescriber. As many as five to ten drug company sales people would visit my office on a given day. How could they spend so much money on promotions, I naively thought? The number of office gifts, each touting their products name and logo, collected on desks, tables, and counters, each one staring at me as if trying to say, "Prescribe me! No me! Hey, doc, over here, prescribe me! I'm better. No, I'm better!" It was ridiculous and getting worse.

So, instead, I asked Ellie, "Would you like to try a pill, patch, cream, or ring?"

She looked puzzled. "Which is better? Umm, which is safer?

I tightened my lips before responding, "I don't know. Ellie. Which sounds the easiest to use?"

She took a deep breath. "I don't know. Guess a pill would be easiest."

"Okay. Let's try a low-dose estrogen tablet."

Defiantly, I wrote for a generic estradiol tablet instead of a brand name. I'm not usually rebellious, but I didn't want to support the drug companies and their powerful influences. The generic would work the same and save the patient an unnecessary expense.

Ellie smiled and thanked me. She would return in one month. I hoped it would help.

When I saw her again, Ellie looked different. Gone was her tired, worried face, now replaced with a healthier looking countenance, a restored twinkle in her eyes.

"Hi, Ellie," I asked although I already knew the answer, "Has the hormone pill helped?"

She nodded. "Yes. I can sleep better, and I'm less anxious during the day. I still have some hot flashes and night sweats, but yes, dealing with home stresses better again. Thank you."

"Good," I thought. "You're up to date with mammograms and your annual PAP smear," I said while reviewing her chart. "So, I'll write for a year's supply. Call if any problems." I paused and smiled. "I'm glad it's helping, Ellie."

Was this the usual scenario for my menopausal patients? No, not always. Some needed higher estrogen doses. And others, who had an intact uterus, needed estrogen as well as a progestin to prevent overstimulation to the endometrium or the lining of the uterus. It wasn't until I took Dr. Rouzier's course that I learned that synthetic progestin was not progesterone. And while it did protect the lining of the uterus, future research demonstrated dangers—a higher risk for heart disease and breast cancer. But I didn't know that at this time. I prescribed what our medical societies recommended, placed trust in their scientific studies supporting the safety of synthetic progestins. From Dr. Rouzier:

> Doctors were on the right track when they determined estrogen replacement needed the counterbalancing effects of its partner hormone. However, they turned to what pharmaceutical companies had to offer: a synthetic progestin called Provera®. Provera® is as unnatural as it gets.
>
> The only health benefit of Provera® is to protect the uterus. This countered by many side effects, as well as risks of heart disease, stroke, breast cancer, or depression. Natural progesterone is just the opposite. It protects against heart disease, stroke, breast cancer, and depression.

A year later, Ellie returned for a routine gynecological exam. I glanced at her vital signs—blood pressure, heart rate, and weight, now twenty pounds heavier than two years ago.

"Hi, Ellie. Still feeling well on the low-dose estrogen pill?

She sighed before speaking. "Well, very few hot flashes or night sweats." She paused before continuing. "But," she paused again "something is not right."

I nodded. "Okay. What's not right, Ellie?"

She stared at the floor. I sensed her uncomfortableness.

"Well, several things," she said, still without eye contact.

"Yes?" I asked, hopefully with a sympathetic and encouraging tone.

She sighed again and made eye contact. "Dr. Birken, I'm a bit embarrassed. I know you're my doctor, but I'm still uncomfortable talking about this."

I knew this was more than her weight gain and guessed it was about libido.

"You know, Paul and I have always enjoyed sex." She looked down again before making eye contact again. "But, I don't seem to want it anymore. And when we do, it hurts! I've never experienced this before."

Not an uncommon complaint. Atrophy, a drying of the vaginal lining along with a decrease in lubrication as well as shrinking of the supporting vaginal structures.

"And," she continued, now more at ease. I keep gaining weight, my sleep is poor, and I can't seem to remember anything." She shook her head. "I feel old, Dr. Birken." She paused. "And I don't like it."

Maybe, I thought, Ellie may be the right person for bio-identical hormones. We have a trusting doctor–patient relationship. Perhaps, she was the person to introduce these concepts.

So, I explained about the recent course I took. The scientific data supporting the use of compounding hormones instead of synthetic, the clinical improvements it could bring as well as the long-term safety. The need to check all hormones, not just the recommended ones to determine if she was menopausal—gonadotropins called FSH (follicular stimulating hormone) and LH (luteinizing stimulating hormone); I already knew she was menopausal, but estradiol, progesterone, thyroid, DHEA (an adrenal hormone that decreases with age), and her testosterone levels—hormone testing never discussed in my conventional teachings, levels that would allow me to individualize a protocol for Ellie and, hopefully, improve her concerns.

Attentively, she listened to my discussion, nodding periodically, absorbed in the details.

"Okay," she said, although I was concerned that it may have been overwhelming, or too emphatic. This was my first patient introduction. Little did I know that within a few years, 90 percent of my medical practice would be devoted to bio-identical hormone optimization, not only for women of all ages but for men as well. "Yes, I want to try these hormones," she continued, appearing excited. "If it would help me with my problems, low sex drive, mental fog, poor sleep, and even with my weight, then yes, it's worth a try."

And I was excited as well but with some uncertainty. Could it help her? I didn't know. But I did agree with Ellie. It was worth a try.

A week later, Ellie sat across from my desk as we reviewed her labs, slowly and thoroughly. She seemed to understand the many details. Her low estradiol, progesterone, and testosterone levels were expected, but Dr. Rouzier taught me how to look deeper into thyroid function testing, more than the recommended screening. Included in the thyroid panel was the "free" or active levels of two thyroid values, T3 and T4, not just the thyroid stimulating hormone (TSH) from the pituitary. I had been taught in the past that the TSH was the determining lab test for an underactive/overactive thyroid. Now I had a more thorough analysis, evaluating thyroid function in a different way; to detect a subtle cause of thyroid insensitivity that many patients experience with age. Dr. Rouzier:

The body makes less and less T3 as we get older. Almost all women over 50 will have free T3 levels in the lower 15th percent of normal. This is due to the fact the body converts less and less T4 to T3.

It is my custom, then and now, to give each patient a copy of their labs to read while I look at my computer screen version, a way to demonstrate all hormone levels and to indicate what is optimal, not the "within normal limits" values, a poor interpretation of lab tests. Unfortunately, when lab companies indicate "normal" values for tests, they are actually using reference ranges, meaning that 98 percent of patients fall between these values. Why are they referred to as "within normal limits?" Who decided that these numbers were "normal?" And yet, physicians use these reference ranges to tell patients that their tests are "normal" when for most, they're not optimal. If hormone values are not in the higher range, then patients may experience the myriad symptoms related to low hormones—fatigue, weight gain, poor sleep, lowered libido, mental fog, and aches and pains. Optimize these levels with bio-identical hormones, and for many, significant clinical improvement occurs. Again, Dr. Rouzier:

> Another important point is the difference between optimal and normal. Normal for one's age is not optimal for one's age.
>
> The medical literature supports replacement levels to that of a younger age, typically 20–30 years old. at these levels, optimal health is attained, as well as the feel-good effects.

I will contest the definition of "normal." I will argue that conservative doctors and ethicists do more harm than good. Optimal hormone therapy, or more correctly termed "preventive" medicine, is about more than just vanity; it is our health and quality of life.

Ellie listened intently, focused on the printed lab values, making notes and nodding in agreement with my interpretations. She put her pen down and looked up.

"I've never understood the importance of hormones. Why has no other doctor discussed this with me before?"

A typical response.

"Ellie," I said, "that's how I was taught. Now I know differently."

Ellie understood this concept—"within normal limits" is a poorly defined parameter and not optimal.

She smiled. "Let's continue please."

And so we did. I discussed her low DHEA levels, an adrenal hormone that decreases with age. Dr. Rouzier:

DHEA is one of the best, if not prime, example of a bioidentical marker for chronological age. As far as longevity is concerned, this was address in *The New England Journal of Medicine* which stated overall morbidity and mortality is directly related to the level of DHEA. High levels of DHEA are associated with increased longevity, whereas low DHEA levels are predictive of early morbidity.

This hormone is very beneficial to health and well-being.

Ellie seemed to understand her labs, what was considered optimal, and which ones correlated with her symptoms. Now the hard part—how to customize a protocol right for her with the understanding that her dosing would probably require tweaking depending on clinical response and the follow-up lab values?

Together, Ellie and I formulated a protocol: low-dose thyroid in the morning, followed by a low-dose bioidentical estrogen capsule, vitamin D and DHEA supplementation, with a combination of estrogen and natural progesterone before bed. Natural progesterone helps with sleep as well as provides protection to the breasts and bones. Dr. Rouzier:

> Progesterone works with estrogen to relieve menopausal symptoms, protect against breast and uterine cancer, and enhance overall feelings of well-being. For pre-menopausal women, progesterone eliminates painful menstrual cramps, mood swings, heavy bleeding, dysphoria, bloating, and menstrual migraines. Natural progesterone has no harmful side effects. If taken in oral form, it can cause some sleepiness.

The testosterone prescription was trickier, not well absorbed orally (although today we have a compounded micronized capsule with good clinical success) and sub-cutaneous pellets that provide the most consistent and balanced delivery of hormones. But at this time, we were limited to two methods only—creams twice per day or the weekly injections, something most women shied from. Ellie chose the creams.

Fortunately, I have an excellent compounding pharmacy near my office—pharmacists who understand bio-identical concepts and who customize compounds based on my recommendations, not like the "one-size-fits-all" approach from the pharmaceutical companies. When I first started, there were few compounders available, but now there are several hundred. Jasper and Keisha Lovoi, husband and wife pharmacists, own and operate The Woodlands Compounding Pharmacy, dedicated to their profession and devoted to making quality compounds. For clinicians, it's important to have a good working relationship with your specialized pharmacist, one who can create unique, individualized products such as capsules, creams, injections, and sublingual bio-identical hormones. Together, the Lovoi's and I brainstorm compounding formulations, protocols, unique for each patient based on clinical presentation, lab tests, and patient compliance. A good relationship is essential between physician and compounding pharmacist.

Ellie stopped her synthetic hormones and started our compounded formulation. I asked her to call with any problems or questions. Three weeks later, one of my nurses would call as a follow-up, today replaced by emails.

It was lunch time, although my scheduled one hour break was now only ten minutes due to a longer than expected surgery. My nurse walked in to my office.

I was staring at a medical journal while wolfing down a microwaved lunch.

"You asked me to call Ellie and I spoke with her today," she said.

I sat up in my chair. "Ellie. Well…well, how's she feeling?"

Casually, my nurse continued, "Oh, she said she feels good."

"Well, what exactly did she mean?"

My nurse made eye contact with me, realizing that my interest was more than perfunctory. "She said she just feels well."

"Did she give you specifics? Sleep, energy?"

My nurse smiled, puzzled by my rapid questioning. "What's going on? Why so interested?"

I sighed and smiled. "She's our first bio-identical hormone patient."

"Oh, I see." She cocked her head to the side. "I didn't ask. Sorry. Didn't know. Thought you just wanted an update on her current estradiol."

My staff knew I was excited to begin evaluating patients for bio-identical hormones. My enthusiasm for the first Dr. Rouzier course was obvious. But, as a typical office day goes, I hadn't told anyone that Ellie was the first patient.

"You know," she said, "it will be interesting to see how she feels." She winked before continuing. "Who knows? Maybe I'll want to try them!"

And yes, within a few months, my staff and my wife were on bio-identical hormones. At the six-week review, Ellie's levels were dramatically improved. Her estradiol, progesterone, testosterone, DHEA, thyroid, and vitamin D levels were now optimal. And it showed in her face.

"Dr. Birken," she said enthusiastically, "I can't believe the changes! I sleep like a baby, have tremendous energy during the day. Mental fog is gone, I have less aches and pains when I wake up, and best of all, I lost six pounds!"

"Great, Ellie," I was ecstatic. My first patient and successful as well. Everything I studied, all the medical journal articles, the hours spent with the compounding pharmacist—all worth it just to hear Ellie's success. I smiled but was afraid to ask about one other problem, her libido. But Ellie continued.

"And you know," she said sheepishly, "our sex lives..." She paused and stared down with embarrassment. "Well, it's like Paul and I are newlyweds again."

It wasn't long before Paul asked to have his labs checked. Not surprising. Yet, I was hesitant as a gynecologist to treat men. Could I? Should I? Why not, I thought? And the trend continued as many other husbands or male partners of my patients called requesting lab reviews for possible bio-identical hormones, a pattern that persists today.

Eventually, several years later, when we began offering subcutaneous pellets for hormones, both Ellie and Paul converted to this method. Pellets provide a consistent and balanced hormone delivery system. Ellie and Paul are just two of the several thousand patients who have chosen hormone pellet insertion. As a couple, they found their vitality and overall sense of well-being, maintaining low body fat, mental clarity, youthfulness, as well as a healthy sex life. From Dr. Donovitz:

> To all the naysayers, to all the physicians who, if they are not up on something they are down on it, to all the academic teachers in our medical schools who have shunned bio-identical hormone optimization and to the insurance companies who believe hormone pellet therapy is experimental, the evidence of efficacy, purity, sterility, and the amazing long-term side-effect profile to the value of this therapy to men and women. Those men and women who want to age healthier, live happier, and have more productive lives should demand that their hormones be evaluated before they are randomly overmedicated for diseases they do not have.

Ellie was our first patient, and we are grateful that she was receptive to an alternative to synthetic hormones and most importantly, her response. From accepting the vicissitudes of aging to embracing medical concepts, not only to improve her quality of life but to reduce her risks for age-related diseases. Ellie validated all that I learned, and helped ignite changes in my practice, a new medical approach toward healthy living. That's where it all started. And because of Ellie, my medical practice moved from treating problems to improving lifestyle and reducing age-related changes, changes that make us feel and look old.

3

Todd

Male andropause can begin any time after age thirty-five.

Each year thereafter, men lose between one and five percent of their testosterone production.

That means on the average, men lose twenty percent of their testosterone per decade. Many lose it much more quickly.

GARY DONOVITZ, MD, PRESIDENT AND FOUNDER
OF BIOTE MEDICAL

For over twenty-five years, I saw female patients for gyne-cologic issues. Now, my physician skills would need adjustments for male patients—different communication techniques, focuses, and concerns—a learning experience. Not since my graduation from medical school in 1976 had I seen a male as a patient. Yes, I had discussions with husbands/male partners regarding surgical outcomes while a patient was in the recovery room, but never with a male as my patient. Maybe it was partly me—a slight uncertainty about my interaction and some doubt reading their body language. Would my dialogue be as effective? Would a male sense my unfamiliarity? How ironic that me, a man, would even doubt my ability to interact with a male patient.

Todd was the husband of Cindy, a longtime patient who had significant clinical success with bio-identical hormone optimization. Todd wanted to have that same vitality and sense of well-being as his wife. A healthy fifty-two-year-old who, over the past three to five years, was now experiencing fatigue, poor sleep, weight gain, especially in the belly, lowered libido and sexual performance, along with mental fog and more aches and pains. But discovering these problems was different with Todd compared to his wife—men are a different animal.

Typically, when I read a patient's medical history, there is much detail regarding symptoms, previous medical problems, and family medical history—but that's with females. Now, with Todd's history, symptoms and medical history were simply left blank. What, I thought? Where was the information I needed to determine a hormone protocol?

Todd sat across my desk looking calm and casual and then smiled.

"You know, Doc, it feels weird being here with all these women in the waiting room."

I never thought about a male patient being uncomfortable in a gynecology office. Yes, I have had males accompany their wives or significant others when making recommendations for gynecological treatments, but not as the actual patient.

"Todd, remember you're here as a patient to discuss hormones." I paused before making a joke, "No PAP smear for you today!"

That broke the proverbial ice. We both laughed and went on with our consultation. But finding out about Todd's problems was like pulling teeth.

"What symptoms are you experiencing, Todd?" I asked, feeling more comfortable with my interaction.

He laughed. "Not sure, Doc. I guess my wife wanted me to come in."

Over the next eighteen years, I would hear similar responses. No doubt about it, most men downplayed their symptoms.

My approach with men is more direct. After the usual denial of problems, I'd ask specific questions regarding fatigue, sleep, weight gain, mental fog, aches and pains, and lowered libido. After a year of treating males, I realized that libido and sexual performance was more than a selfish concern, it was an issue revolving around their manhood, an instinct needed for survival of the species.

Eventually, Todd admitted to everything—twenty pounds of weight gain, struggles with energy, erratic sleep, increased pain with physical activity, mental fog, and of course, reduced libido. I knew that low testosterone contributed to all these symptoms, except one that I didn't know about—a decrease in motivation and drive, another male concern.

"You know, Doc," Todd continued, "I just lost my mojo." Todd twisted his lips. He paused before continuing, "I don't have that drive any more. Used to look forward to work, but now I go just because I have to. Not like me. Not like me at all."

A problem that I never gave much consideration to before. And when I think about myself, before optimizing my testosterone, I struggled with multitasking, but yes, perhaps a decrease in motivation. Once my levels were good, I did rediscover that lost drive—to learn and apply myself further. I remained dedicated to providing the best care for my patients, but I was more complacent about personal goals—my workouts and especially my tenacity and "push"—a characteristic that I had cherished—an ambition to succeed professionally and personally. I understood Todd.

After reviewing his labs, Todd's symptoms were obviously hormonal. Low vitamin D, suboptimal thyroid and DHEA, and most importantly, low testosterone.

Todd nodded as I explained every lab result. He looked up before speaking. "You know, Doc, I had my primary care physician check my testosterone level about three years ago and he told me I was in the normal range."

Again, another misguided interpretation. Not the doctor's fault, but a product of not understanding optimal values. From Dr. Donovitz:

Testosterone levels are at their highest during adolescence and early adulthood. The normal range of testosterone levels in healthy males is between 800–1200 nanograms per decliter (ng/Dl). After age thirty, testosterone levels in men decline—sometimes precipitously.

Todd's testosterone level was 390. Most labs list the "normal" range (98 percent of all male levels) between approximately 350 and 1,200. The testosterone level collected by his family doctor was 475, and hence was told he was normal. Todd had low "T" and needed help. In addition, his free testosterone was low. Most physicians don't check this, which is unfortunate. Several men have come to my practice with close to optimal total testosterone levels but with low free testosterone, which creates symptoms of low T. But what is free testosterone? Dr. Rouzier:

Much of a man's testosterone is tied up or bound to a protein called sex hormone binding globulin

(SHBG). Research has shown that free testosterone becomes more bound with age, leaving readily available testosterone low while total testosterone remains high. It is the fall in bio-available or free testosterone that is responsible for the signs and symptoms or andropause.

Todd understood my explanations regarding lab results as well as clinical correlation and was ready to start hormone optimization. We discussed boosting his thyroid with a biological thyroid capsule in the morning, adding pharmaceutical-grade vitamin D3 and DHEA, and starting testosterone. At this time in my bio-identical career, we only had two types of testosterone treatments, creams and weekly injections. Todd was unsure—he didn't like needles but questioned the use of topical medications. I explained that *commercially* made testosterone cream was synthetic, weak, and very expensive, while *compounded* testosterone cream was bio-identical, stronger, and significantly more economical, again confirming the additional cost created by the pharmaceutical industry. He decided to try creams but had another worry.

"Dr. Birken, my father had prostate cancer. Should I be concern about starting testosterone?"

I smiled. Todd had failed to list this under family medical history, so typical of men. I explained the lack of scientific data regarding testosterone use and prostate cancer. Dr. Abram Morgentaler, the director of Men's Health Boston and associate clinical professor of urology at *Harvard Medical School*, Beth Israel Deaconess Medical Center, has done extensive research on testosterone effects on the prostate:

> Prostate cancer becomes more prevalent in men as they age, and that's also when their testosterone levels decline. We almost never see it in men in their peak testosterone years, in their 20s for instance. We know from autopsy studies that 8% of men in their 20s already have tiny prostate cancers, so if testosterone really made prostate cancer grow so rapidly—we used to talk about it like it was pouring gasoline on a fire—we should see some appreciable rate of prostate cancer in men in their 20s. We don't. So, I'm no longer worried that giving testosterone to men will make their hidden cancer grow, because I'm convinced that it doesn't happen.

Todd was reassured. I prescribed a compounded testosterone cream to be applied twice per day but not before bed since it could transfer to his wife. Todd was to call if any problems with repeat labs in six weeks.

Three weeks later, I emailed Todd regarding his clinical response to the hormones. Typically, he replied with a common patient comment—surprised that a physician would take the time to send an email. Unfortunately, medical care has become diluted and more impersonal. But why? Was it the nature of new physicians today? I didn't think so. Probably a combination of many factors: poor insurance reimbursements, malpractice constraints, and the need to see more patients in order to pay for office staff, rent, phones, and the high annual fee for liability insurance. It took a leap of faith for me to go "out of network" with medical insurance companies. My fees were reasonable and it lifted the restraints on my medical care, and more importantly, the need to hurry my patient visits.

Now I could spend close to an hour with new patients and at least thirty minutes for follow-up visits, a luxury compared to the previous need to see patients every five minutes. After twenty years in practice, my office visits and surgical reimbursements were less than when I had started practice in 1980. When I called the usual insurance players—United, Blue Cross/Blue Shield, Humana, Cigna, and so on, the response was the same—nothing we can do from our end, you just need to see more patients. Outlandish! Like the proverbial hand choke, the insurance companies and personal injury attorneys were slowly strangulated the art of medicine. No wonder doctors, as well as patients, were becoming disillusioned with current medical care. Todd's email:

Hi Dr. Birken! Thanks for the email. I have more energy during the day. Like that! But, no change in libido and still have my aches and pains. And no weight loss although I am working out more now.

Thanks again for the email! Looking forward to see my next set of labs in 3 weeks.

Todd

Hmm, I thought. Todd's DHEA, vitamin D, and thyroid were probably helping with energy but the testosterone cream was not being well absorbed, a common problem with creams.

At six weeks, the office called Todd as a reminder to recheck his hormone levels, and as suspected, his thyroid, DHEA, and vitamin D were much improved, but his total and free testosterone levels were minimally elevated.

"Todd, you're not absorbing the cream well. Would you consider weekly injections?"

Todd squirmed in his seat. "Doc, I don't know why but I hate needles."

I nodded. "Could Cindy give you the injection?"

He rubbed his chin. "Don't know. I'll ask her."

"The other option," I said, "is to come to our office weekly and have one of my nurses give you the shot."

"Okay," he responded. "I'll ask Cindy first."

Not surprisingly, Cindy had no problems administering the injection. I have a patient who taught his thirteen-year-old daughter to give him the shot! Testosterone is administered intramuscularly, but the compounded solution, compared to commercial made testosterone, is thinner, more aqueous, and is given with a small needle. I prescribed Todd a combination of both a short-acting and long-acting testosterone solution that would provide a more consistent level throughout the week, unlike the thicker, more painful, and long-acting only commercially made product, another credit to working with compounding pharmacists who can customized prescriptions according to the patients' needs and not for the drug company's profitability. And while testosterone injections are not bio-identical, prescribed in a judicious manner with careful lab testing every six months, not only improve quality of life, but afford long-term benefits as well. I emailed

Todd four weeks later. He replied:

Hi Dr. Birken,
    The shots are going very well.
    No problem with Cindy giving it to me weekly. And I feel great! Libido is like when I was teenager. No more aches and pains. Want to work out now. And best of all, I've lost 8 pounds and my waist size has dropped two sizes!
    This is wonderful!

A nice email to read. Not unlike most doctors, I wanted to hear positive results from my patients and this one made my day. There was one more line in the email.

> By the way, Doc, Cindy looks forward to giving me the injection.
>> I just need to be nice to her on "shot" day!
>> Thanks for everything.
>> Todd

I smiled not realizing how often I would hear or read this comment. Eventually, Todd changed to subcutaneous pellet insertions when I started offering this service, lasting six months and providing consistent and balanced testosterone levels. Todd lost a total of twenty pounds, his waist went from thirty-six to thirty-one inches, and his cholesterol level dropped over a hundred points within six months of starting hormones. Another success. But more importantly, both Cindy and Todd were happy— not only with their clinical improvements, but with both embracing a more vibrant and healthy lifestyle.

The transition from seeing women only to seeing both sexes was smoother than I anticipated, and helping both women and men, especially couples, is most gratifying to me as a physician. Best of all, I could relate to the men I saw as patients now that my testosterone was optimized. Once I started thyroid and testosterone, my life changed both physically and emotionally. No more fatigue, reduced aches and pains, and especially a new zeal for the gifts of life. My body fat dropped from 28 to 14 percent and my waist reduced from thirty-six to thirty-one. And no more Lipitor—my cholesterol dropped over a hundred points. Yes, it was easy for me to identify with these men and my story added credence to their symptoms as well.

In the future, more and more couples would seek hormone optimization, to benefit individually and for the relationship as well. These couples now had restored vitality, a refreshed bonding, and most importantly, a rejuvenated life, individually as well as together.

4

Angie

Testosterone as the "male hormone" is a misnomer. Testosterone is just as much a female hormone. If anyone tells you differently, they have not studied their general human biology. Society as a whole feels safer when things are in compartments: estrogen is a female hormone; testosterone is a male hormone, thus the uproar and obstinacy over testosterone supplementation in women.

DR. NEAL ROUZIER

For many female patients, an annual gynecological exam is more than a necessity, and perhaps, a burdensome preventive health requirement. When you've been in practice as long as I have, some patients become "friends"—those who have shared pregnancies, health issues such as heart disease, surgeries, and even cancers; more importantly, major life changes—career changes, divorces, family deaths, and the many sundry vicissitudes of life. So an annual exam was also a visit, a time to "catch up" on a patient's life, the cherished relationship between a doctor and patient. Angie was one of those.

First seen when she was newly married at twenty-five years, Angie's "history" included two healthy pregnancies and a surgery for a ruptured ovarian cyst. Unfortunately, at the age of forty-two, her husband filed for a divorce, a devastating event for a woman who had married for life. It took her two years to adjust—sadness turning into depression requiring psychotherapy and "mood" medication to help with sleep and her "blues." But, like many patients, she was able to climb out of her lows while becoming strongly independent and starting a successful home business based on hard work, dedication, and focus. Angie had to adjust to her life changes. And instead of becoming bitter and angry at the loss of her marriage, she blossomed with a new attitude, free of victimization.

I was proud of her. Many of my patients wallowed in self-pity, remaining unhappy, and especially, angry at their ex-spouses—a negative intimacy that sustained them, compromising personal advancement. But not Angie. At the age of forty-eight years, she now faced a new obstacle—one that was physiologic rather than circumstantial.

"How have you been, Angie?" I asked cheerfully, expecting to see a friendly smile.

Her look was different. She sighed and lower her head, not what I expected. "Dr. Birken, I'm having problems." I waited before she made eye contact and continued, "I think I need help." She swallowed. "I...I'm tired, gaining weight, and can't sleep."

And she did appear tired. I noticed more facial wrinkles then the year before. "How long have you felt this way?" I asked.

"Oh, about six to nine months. But"—she paused again—"I'm having another problem."

Usually, I let the patient continue with her complaints. But this was so uncharacteristic for Angie that I felt a need to encourage her. "Go ahead, Angie. What other problem?" I asked but had a suspicion. When patients are reticent, it's usually about libido. Was Angie dating?

"Dr. Birken," she continued, "I met someone."

Yes, I thought. I was right.

"And, you know, I wasn't ready for this."

"Ready for what, Angie?"

"Well, to become sexually active again." She paused again, looking pensive before continuing, "I didn't expect it to happen. But it did."

For most patients, this was a difficult issue to discuss— but when someone trusts their doctor, it's easier to talk about intimacy problems.

"You know, I like this guy. He's very caring, respectful… all the things you want from a man. But…" She sighed again. "I don't seem to want to have sex." She smiled. "There, I said it. That wasn't easy."

Situations like this one can be very uncomfortable for patients, and yet for others, not. But I was glad that she felt secure enough to share her concerns.

"Angie, there are many factors for low libido. You've done so well with your life after your divorce. But still, there are emotional factors that may be causing this."

She nodded. "Yes, but here's the twist. I like him. And I feel something for him. But not just the lack of libido." She looked down before continuing, "When we make love…it hurts." I never experienced this when I was married."

Yes, there was more than psychology here. Now I needed to ask questions.

"Angie, do have you have night sweats?"

"Yes, I do. How did you know?"

"Vaginal dryness?"

"Yes."

"Bladder problems, like urgency and frequency, maybe losing urine? And your periods? Are they erratic?"

Her eyes widened. "Yes. All of that." She appeared more worrisome. "What's wrong? How did you know this?"

I wasn't clairvoyant. These were symptoms related to perimenopause. A time in a woman's life when hormones changed. The ovaries still worked, just not as well. Testosterone, progesterone, and thyroid levels fall. Menstrual cycles can become more frequent or even infrequent and occasionally heavy with episodes of spotting. There's weight gain, night sweats, and daytime fatigue. Usually, hot flashes are not an issue since the patient may be estrogen dominant, where ovarian activity can produce estrogen surges, resulting in bloating, breast tenderness, and weight gain. Some women don't complain of vaginal dryness, but in Angie's case, her occasionally low estrogen levels were causing vaginal atrophy, hence the dryness and especially the bladder issues since the uro-epithelium, the lining to the urethra and bladder, are highly dependent on proper hormone levels. Angie had classic perimenopausal symptoms and needed help. Sadly, as a gynecologist, we are taught to prescribe a low-dose birth control pill, something promoted by the pharmaceutical industry. But as I learned to optimize hormones with bio-identical hormones, I realized that the pill only regulated cycles but did nothing for the other problems. Or, if the patient didn't want to take "the pill" or had a medical contraindication, I would recommend Prozac or a similar antidepressant, a drug that did little and usually created more problems, especially with libido and weight. For years, I remained angry at the drug companies before I finally let go, now grateful for the new knowledge to treat patients effectively. Sadly, most physicians today still treat perimenopausal women the same way. A reviewer writes about Suzanne Somers's book, *I'm Too Young for This!*

> She explains that perimenopause is the most dangerous phase for women because of the significant fluctuation of their hormones. "You go through puberty and the blissful days of your 20s, and then things start to change. The mood in the house starts to change, and one day you wake up and you and your husband don't recognize the person you've become." She adds that the symptoms you experience are your body screaming, "All is not well!"

Angie had her labs collected. Ten days later, we reviewed her results. As predicted, her thyroid levels were suboptimal, hence the fatigue and weight gain; her estrogen was high and progesterone low, although I knew at times her estrogen levels would be significantly low causing vaginal atrophy. Most critically, her testosterone level was extremely low, hence low libido and compromised sexual response. Angie understood my explanations and was excited to try bio-identical hormones. We discussed options and agreed on the following protocol:

1. Low-dose biological thyroid in the morning on an empty stomach.
2. Progesterone, orally, before bed.
3. Testosterone cream, applied twice per day.
4. An over-the-counter product that contains a combination of diindolylmethane and indole 3 carbinol derived from plant substances contained in "cruciferous" vegetables such as cabbage, brussels sprouts, cauliflower, and broccoli. Scientist have found that these compounds alter estrogen metabolism in both men and women, possible protecting against hormone-dependent cancers such as those of the breast, cervix, and prostate.

Again from the reviewer on Suzanne Somers's book:

Targeting women 35–50, the book describes in great detail why we may experience unexplained symptoms like weight gain, irritability, insomnia, and decreased sex drive at this age, and provides natural options for hormonal balance through diet, supplementation, healthy practices like getting adequate sleep and exercise, and BHRT (bio-identical hormones).

Again, my protocol is to follow up with the patient by email in three weeks and to repeat labs at six weeks. Of course, any problems would necessitate changes or labs sooner. Angie responded:

Hi Doctor Birken!

Thanks for the email. I can tell things are changing. Not dramatic, but better. Energy, sleep and especially my bladder—much improved!

However, my libido may be a bit higher but still off.

Thanks again for the email. Curious to see what my next of labs show.

Angie.

First email responses vary—most patients don't send a reply, but some are very detailed while others are terse, one or two sentences. Yet, most are positive regarding the clinical response to bio-identical hormones. Angie was a mixed report—some symptoms improved, others did not. We would wait until her next set of labs.

When Angie arrived for her second visit, she looked better—her smile was back and skin was more radiant, a change I could detect immediately. And her labs were better—thyroid was now optimal as well as progesterone level. While her total testosterone was much improved, her free testosterone, or active, bio-available level, was still low. Why? Another perimenopausal problem best explained by her ovarian estrogen level. When high, so was her sex hormone binding globulin, a protein neatly abbreviated as SHBG, which when high, binds to testosterone and makes it less active. From Dr. Rouzier:

> Endocrinologists did not believe testosterone took a dip after 45, because they were measuring the wrong type of testosterone. They measured the total amount of testosterone rather than focusing on free testosterone. Only when doctors and scientist honed in on the bioavailable testosterone did they realize there was a definite decline.

Angie and I had already discussed injections instead of creams. If I had subcutaneous pellets available at that time, then that would have been a better choice for her. But we didn't. And Angie had no problem using the creams twice per day. So I made two changes.

"Angie, if we continue with the cream, I want to increase the strength."

Usually, we started at 2 percent or 20 mg per milliliter, but I increased it to 4 percent and had one other recommendation:

"Instead of applying the cream to the inner thigh region, I'm going to ask you to apply it to different region." I paused before continuing. Angie nodded. "I'm going to change the base of the cream and have you apply it to the vaginal opening."

Angie appeared confused. "Why? Why vaginally?"

So I explained that the vaginal tissue, or mucosa, absorbs cream better than the dermis, or inner thigh, due to thinness and better blood supply. Angie nodded in agreement.

"Okay. No problem with that. Let's try it."

Before I could send a follow-up email in three weeks, I received a follow-up from Angie in two weeks:

Dr. Birken,

Just want to let you know that I feel great now! Not only do I have more energy but my libido is back to when I was younger!

I am a little embarrassed writing this, but heck, you're my doctor.

This is wonderful! Thanks and see you in six months.

Angie

Angie continued to do well with her bio-identical hormones. When I saw her six months later, she not only appeared happy but had lost ten pounds. And her new relationship was strong, based on trust and openness.

"You know, Dr. Birken, I didn't realize what kind of relationship I had before. You meet someone and plan to spend the rest of your life with them. But now, I know it wasn't stable when I compare to what I have now."

I was pleased. Angie had a new life.

"And you know, these hormones not only helped me feel better, but I am stronger physically and emotionally," she said, smiling.

And it made sense. When reproductive and metabolic hormones are low, so are the brain hormones, or neurotransmitters. Improvement with moods was an added bonus to hormone optimization. As a physician, it was gratifying to see many patients stop antidepressants, sleeping pills, or attention-deficit medications.

Perimenopause is a challenging hormone episode for some women. Angie continued to do well. Several years later, when she was menopausal, we added natural estradiol to her protocol, a smooth transition for her. She continues to thrive, physically, mentally, socially, and emotionally.

5

Ryan

I have treated patients on the brink of a physical and emotional meltdown who, with the help of hormone replacement therapy, have experienced renewed energy and sense of well-being, nothing short of a miracle. The stories will make anyone wary because of their too-good-to-be-true nature.

DR. NEAL ROUZIER

Shortly after offering hormone optimization, I noticed an unusual pattern—young men, thirty to forty-five years of age—were making appointments. Leary of their motives, I was surprised with my first patient, a thirty-two-year-old car salesman. Ryan looked young, but his affect was old—difficulty focusing during our conversation, and lack of vitality in his speech. First, I thought he wanted testosterone to "bulk up," not an indication for testosterone. But I soon found out that I was wrong. Ryan was struggling and for good reason.

He had a successful career, moving up on the proverbial corporate ladder, but he now faced a physical and emotional roadblock.

"Dr. Birken," he said, almost pleading, "something is wrong with me and a friend of mine saw you and is doing great."

Still suspicious, I nodded in encouragement for him to continue.

"I can't focus. And I'm exhausted. I drink six diet cokes throughout the day and that's after my morning coffee." He looked down. "And, sadly, I have no sex drive." He looked up with a desperate stare. "My wife asked me if it was her. But I told her no. I love her. I love my family, my job." He took a deep breath. "So I told her I was going to see you. My family doctor has run several blood tests on me and tells me I'm healthy…nothing wrong." He paused and swallowed before continuing, "You're my last hope, Dr. Birken."

Ouch, I thought. This guy is telling me the truth or he needs to win an Oscar. But why, I thought, would a thirty-two-year-old man have low testosterone?

"Ryan, it would be unusual for you to have low T at your age." I glanced at his medical history again and saw the typical male answers—"negative"—written for past medical and family history as well as medications. Yes, he had a few alcoholic drinks per week and occasionally had a cigar, but nothing else. "Let's look at your hormone panel together, Ryan," I said, now thinking that a psychiatric referral may be indicated.

We reviewed his comprehensive metabolic panel—blood sugar, kidney function, electrolytes, liver function tests as well as complete blood count. All normal. His T3 thyroid needed some help. While he was not by definition "hypothyroid," he would benefit with a low-dose biological thyroid, but that wouldn't help his libido. I scrolled to the next page. And my eyes widened.

"Ryan, your two testosterone levels, total and free, are very low."

He made eye contact but I couldn't read his facial expression. Shock? Joy? Or a mixture of both?

I continued, "How long have your felt this way?

He leaned toward my desk. "About a year, but you know, maybe it's been longer."

"Have you ever had a head injury? Sports or car accident?"

"No. I played soccer and had my bell rung going for a header...but no...never had a concussion."

The next question was going to be harder, but I had to ask. "Ever taken steroids to bulk up?"

He shook his head. "Never. I had friends who did that but that's not me." His statement sounded convincing.

Hmm? Why did this guy have low testosterone, I thought? Yet, I didn't realize that I would see more men like Ryan in the ensuing years. And I've discussed this with other bioidentical hormone doctors, even Drs. Rouzier and Donovitz, both making the same observation but without an explanation. Nutrition with chemical additives? Toxins in the air and water? Or maybe, doctors didn't check this in the past and many young males went undiagnosed. I knew I needed to investigate further hormones for Ryan, such as pituitary problems and other potential endocrinopathies. But over the past eighteen years, I have not found another reason for low testosterone levels in young men.

Obviously, Ryan was relieved to find an explanation for his symptoms, although concerned that something else was wrong. First, we needed to treat his low levels.

"Ryan," I asked, "are and your wife planning to have more children?"

"Well, not now. We have one child…she's three." He paused and smiled. "And a handful!"

I smiled back as I remembered my days with young children. The nonstop care, focus, involvement, and, of course, normal parental worry. I didn't want to scare Ryan—wait till she becomes a teenager! Now at my age, I have grandchildren. And they are wonderful. One of my brothers-in-law said it best: "You know. Having grand-children is God's gift to you for not killing your kids when they were young!" Yep, I understand that one.

Pensively, Ryan answered, "My wife and I have talked about more children but not just now."

"Okay, Ryan. We could try to increase your testosterone level with human chorionic gonadotropin, or HCG, or con-sider a medication called clomiphene citrate." Ryan nod-ded. "But it doesn't work as well as using testosterone." Now I leaned toward Ryan. "But, it can lower your sperm count." I paused to allow Ryan time to take this all in. "But, if you and your wife want to attempt conception, then you'll have to come off the testosterone and try a different method, one that will not compromise your fertility."

He nodded. "I understand, Dr. Birken, and I appreciate the options." He sighed. "But right now, I don't think I could impregnate my wife even if we wanted to."

I felt sorry for Ryan. His low testosterone levels were significant and affecting his career, marriage, parenting, and personal confidence. But there was more to be con-cerned about. From Dr. Donovitz:

> Over the long term, men with low testosterone have an increased risk for heart disease, stroke,

diabetes, Alzheimer's, prostate cancer, arthritis, osteoporosis, and muscle loss.

Ryan and I discussed options for testosterone use. He was concerned about using creams—transference to his wife and daughter, and wasn't sure about pellets, although the concept for continuous and consistent testosterone levels over six months was appealing to him. After considering the options, he elected to give himself a weekly injection, although slightly squeamish about needles. I optimized his thyroid and started him on DHEA and vitamin D. Six weeks later, he was sitting across my desk, a different look, and especially, a new attitude, evident by his broad smile and assertive handshake.

"How are you feeling, Ryan?" I asked, although I already knew the answer.

"Great! Can't believe the difference," he said with confidence, the antithesis to the personality I met six weeks ago. "Dr. Birken, this is what I needed! Everything has changed." He paused before continuing, with what I thought was a slightly mischievous smile. "And my wife can't believe the difference either." Again, a pause. "She told me to tell you that I need less testosterone!" he said now with an almost imperceptible wink, a universal male sign indicating, I'm having a lot of sex, know what I mean?

And his repeat labs were perfect. Both total and free testosterone levels were optimal as well as thyroid, DHEA, and Vitamin D.

"Any problems with the injection, Ryan?"

"Well, yes, at first. Didn't like to stick myself, but heck, I'll take a little pain for the benefits."

Yes, another typical response. But I was happy for Ryan. His life was different. And for a young male, a renewal, not only physically, but emotionally—confident and content, a revived self -esteem and motivation.

For the next two years, I saw Ryan every six months. And every time, Ryan validated the need for hormone optimization, for his marriage, parenting, and career. But that was about to change when he called three months after our last hormone consultation.

"Dr. Birken," he said sheepishly, "Lisa and I have talked and..." He paused. "We're ready to have another child."

This was the first male patient of mine who had reached this decision, although since then, I have had many men who faced this dilemma. Testosterone, although not with every male, reduces sperm production, compromising fertility. Ryan needed to stop his testosterone and allow several months before spermatogenesis created enough viable sperm to impregnate his wife. I would prescribe HCG, or human chorionic gonadotropin, a stimulant to his pituitary allowing his testes to produce more testosterone. Reluctantly, he was ready.

"How different am I going to feel, Dr. Birken?"

"Don't know, Ryan. Some men do well with HCG, but the increase in testosterone is not the same as giving yourself testosterone." Usually, levels would be nominally changed, but it was better than nothing at all.

Ryan nodded and started on HCG injections, now a subcutaneous, allergy needle instead of an intramuscular injection but requiring use every other day. The injections, although simple, would probably provide minimal clinical effect for a man with low testosterone levels. And a month later, I received an email from Ryan.

> Hi Dr. Birken. Hope all is well. Now been about 4 weeks that I stopped the testosterone injections and started the HCG. Not feeling well.
>
> Libido is gone, not good for my wife and I in order to conceive.
>
> I'm tired, sleeping poorly, and have mental fog. Maybe not as bad as when I first came to see you but pretty bad. Anything else I can do?

The responses were the same as I saw more men who switched from testosterone to HCG—clinically, not like testosterone. I asked Ryan to recheck his labs and found his total testosterone barely over five hundred, well below our goal of nine hundred to twelve hundred. His free testosterone, or active/bio-available levels, were slightly better than the initial values. I had Ryan change his HCG to a daily injection as well as increasing the dose. A few weeks later, he emailed again, and noted a marginal improvement. This was the best we could do for Ryan—a testament to the limitations of HCG and improvement of testosterone levels.

Several months later, my receptionist came to my office during my abbreviated lunch break, dwindled from one hour to fifteen minutes, not atypical for a busy day.

"Dr. Birken, Ryan called and wanted to speak with you. He said its important."

I nodded. "Okay," I said as I swallowed a bite from my sandwich. "See if you can get him on the phone before I start seeing afternoon patients."

Leaning back in my chair, I pondered about the conversation and wondered if Ryan and Lisa had given up on having another child. Surely, his low testosterone was taking a toll on him as well as the marriage.

My receptionist interrupted my reverie. "He's on line three."

After one more gulp of water, I reached for the phone. "Hi, Ryan. How are you?" I asked expecting a somber voice at the other end. Surprisingly, it was just the opposite.

"Dr. Birken"—Ryan's voice was loud and reverberating with excitement—"Lisa," he said excitingly, "She's pregnant!"

I smiled. "Wow. Great news, Ryan! How far along is she?"

Like a kid wound up on excitement, Ryan continued, "Umm, don't know. She did a pregnancy test a few hours ago! It's positive." And with just a minimal segue he continued, "Can you order my testosterone shots today?

Silently, I laughed. Yes, Ryan was missing those testosterone benefits. A bit cynically, I wondered if he was more excited about restarting testosterone than his wife's positive pregnancy test! But there was nothing wrong to be excited about both.

A few weeks later, we rechecked his levels, all optimal again and his vitality restored. Lisa's pregnancy was uncomplicated. Now they had two healthy daughters and no plans for more children. Eventually, Ryan chose subcutaneous pellets for the convenience and consistency. After fifteen years, I now see Lisa for her perimenopausal symptoms. Both continue to enjoy their family and youthful lifestyle, another bio-identical success. And to this day, my colleagues and I are still puzzled why we see young males with low testosterone and wonder if it is environmental or a condition that conventional medicine never addressed before. Maybe medical science will discover a reason for low testosterone in young male adults. But there is an urgent need for clinicians to investigate this possibility in these men. As physicians, our training is intense but can be limiting, necessitating continuous medical education, to learn about newer concepts in diagnostic and treatment options.

6

Angela

Insulin resistance appears to be a syndrome that is associated with a clustering of metabolic disorders, including non-insulin-dependent diabetes mellitus, obesity, hypertension, lipid abnormalities, and atherosclerotic cardiovascular disease.

AMERICAN DIABETES ASSOCIATION

Soon, I discovered the most prevalent endocrine or hormone problem among premenopausal women, a condition casually addressed in medical school as well as postgraduate education, not only by gynecologists but internists and endocrinologists as well. Aware of the multiple symptoms and presentations, I now investigate labs that are indicators of a common condition that causes many women problems - insulin resistance (metabolic syndrome), or more commonly referred to, but not quite correctly, as polycystic ovarian syndrome. Dr. Rouzier states that 10 percent of premenopausal women have this genetically induced hormone problem that can lead to weight gain, acne, facial hair, thinning scalp hair, fatigue, infertility, and menstrual irregularities. However, not every woman exhibits all these symptoms. According to Dr. Rouzier:

> Primary defect is hyperinsulinemia with enlarged ovaries with beta cell dysfunction causing insulin resistance and alpha cell dysfunction causing increase in glucagon which increases glucose absorption as well as gluconeogenesis from proteins, fats, and glycogen.

After many years of treating women with this problem, I now understand how to interpret appropriate lab testing, but unfortunately, most clinicians are not aware of its prevalence—a condition, when treated, may help with weight loss, improve energy, reduce acne and facial hair, regulate menstrual cycles, and enhance fertility. Insulin resistance (IR) or polycystic ovarian syndrome (PCOS) patients, appropriately treated, not only feel better but have a reduction in cardiovascular disease, obesity, hypertension, diabetes, fatty liver, and breast as well as uterine cancer. But a physician must be suspicious for its occurrence and understand this altered hormonal/metabolic state.

During one of Dr. Rouzier's intensive training sessions when he spent considerable time discussing IR and PCOS, I realized how many patients I had seen with this condition but was unaware of its diagnosis. Ironically, my training as an obstetrician/gynecologist emphasized irregular menstrual cycles, possible infertility, and multicystic ovarian findings on ultrasound but not the significant underling endocrine problems—a genetic disposition where a patient's pancreas produces more insulin than the body needs. Not every woman exhibits all these conditions—some have acne and no weight gain, others have weight gain and no acne and yet others have only menstrual irregularities/infertility, multisymptom pathology with individual clinical expressions.

Angela was an established patient of mine; I had birthed her youngest child and was subsequently providing gynecological care for many years thereafter. Always cheerful and appreciative, Angela was a delight to see yearly, conscientious about her health, never missing a PAP smear or mammogram. However, her menstrual history was significant—irregular and heavy. Exams and even ultrasounds were negative (some patients do not show enlarged, cystic ovaries with sonograms). Angela tried a low-dose pill but had side effects—bloating, weight gain, poor sleep, lowered libido. She continued to have unpredictable menstrual cycles, some heavy and painful, but she didn't complain and accepted this as part of her life. But at age forty-seven, things changed. Her cycles were just as erratic, but symptoms of fatigue and especially weight gain remained—she had gained almost twenty pounds in the last two years although she ate clean and exercised five days a week.

"I don't get it," she said during her appointment. "I practically starve myself and do an hour of hard cardio." She shook her head. "My husband eats anything and never gains weight. Not fair!"

She asked to have her hormones checked. We spent considerable time discussing her suboptimal thyroid and low progesterone levels, but one test stood out— her follicular stimulating hormone (FSH) and luteinizing hormone (LS). Produced by the pituitary gland, FSH and LH stimulate ovarian activity, a delicate hormone dance that allows proper estrogen and progesterone production, and more importantly, the precise timing to ovulate for conception. As a physician, I found that the many hormone variables so complex—a balanced coordination from the hypothalamus and pituitary in the brain to the ovaries and its hormone production, perfectly timed between an egg and a sperm and the receptivity of uterine lining for implantation of a fertilized egg—that I wondered how a woman ever conceived! But our anatomy and physiology work well together, a magnificent orchestration, allowing our species to reproduce and to survive.

"Angela," I said in a nonalarming way, but upfront and honestly, "I have a concern about a condition that is common." I smiled reassuringly. "Matter of fact..."

I paused and then continued, "you may have had this most of your reproductive years."

Angela, obviously, appeared surprise. "My whole reproductive years," she pondered. "Not sure I understand, Dr. Birken."

I expected this response and went on to explain about IR, qualifying my discussion with the need to confirm my clinical suspicions.

"Angela, I have been looking for this in patients for the past few years. Until I learned how to diagnose it, I believe that I, and many other physicians, were not looking for it."

Angela nodded, and appropriately, inquired what else was necessary.

"I need to repeat blood work, but this time, with you fasting. I want to look at two more tests—insulin and hemoglobin A1C."

It has many names—glycated hemoglobin, glycohemoglobin, glycosylated hemoglobin, a means of determining the average blood sugar concentrations for the preceding three to four months. Most women have elevated fasting insulin levels as well. Usually, there is a reversal in the ratio of FHS to LH. The adrenal hormone called DHEA-S may be elevated as well. But a clinician has to piece together the patients' symptoms with the labs.

Angela's initial tests indicated reversed FSH/LH level, elevated DHEA-Sulfate, as well as an elevated free testosterone level, while her total testosterone was normal. Why the elevated bio-available testosterone? Again, a reduction in sex hormone binding globulin from the liver, allowing more testosterone to be active, and hence the acne, facial hair, and thinning scalp hair. But the increased insulin is a major metabolic problem causing the body to store fat, especially in the abdomen. And with insult to injury, the patient has carbohydrate cravings, making it more difficult to diet. Sadly, many obese patients produce more insulin compounding their weight issues. In addition, Angela's lipid profile was abnormal, elevated cholesterol and especially her LDL or "bad" cholesterol.

"Dr. Birken, I can't eat any healthier!" She sighed before continuing, "And I'm worried. My maternal grandmother developed diabetes when she was in her sixties. And my dad had a heart attack when he was in his late fifties."

Yes, all concerns. But I needed that fasting insulin and hemoglobin A1C level to confirm my suspicions. A week later, the results were back.

Angela returned to the office for the review. I could tell she was anxious about the results, frustrated with her weight struggles, longing for an answer.

"Angela. Your fasting insulin level is at the upper limits of the normal range."

She frowned with disappointment. But I needed to expand the discussion.

"However, according to many medical studies, it's too high."

She looked surprised.

"Again," I continued, "these are references ranges. Most doctors assume they're normal." I paused. "Your level is at twenty-one. The lab states normal values are from two to twenty-five. But it's too high. It needs to be in the single digits. And your hemoglobin A1C is slightly elevated at five point nine. I'd like to see that under five point six."

Angela sat back in her chair, absorbing the information. I could tell she felt relieved but also concerned. I was right.

"Dr. Birken, okay, so now I have insulin resistance. But how do we treat it?"

"Yes, Angela, now that we know your condition, we need to discuss options."

Usually, I would talk about the diet recommendations, especially a low glycemic diet, and exercise, but Angela was already eating this way and worked out regularly. The next step was medication. The hallmark drug is metformin, a commonly prescribed medication for the treatment of type 2 diabetes mellitus that works by increasing peripheral glucose uptake and utilization as well as decreasing hepatic gluconeogenesis. In more simplistic terms, metformin helps control the amount of sugar in the blood, decreases the amount of glucose absorbed from food, and the amount of glucose made by the liver. Metformin also increases the body's response to insulin, a natural substance controlling the amount of glucose in the blood. And recently, there have been studies indicating other health benefits: research suggesting that metformin may slow the aging process and increase lifespan. Metformin has been shown to have anticancer and anti-cardiovascular disease benefits and can also reduce a prediabetic's chance of developing the disease by a third. Interestingly, there are other medications called glucagon-like peptide receptor agonists or GLP-1 agonist. Given subcutaneously, the mechanism by which GLP-1 receptor agonists induce weight loss is believed to be related to multiple actions with the brain and gastrointestinal tract as well as a reduction in hunger. However, they are very expensive, while metformin is not.

Angela listened to my discussion, especially the potential gastrointestinal side effects and the need to monitor fasting insulin, hemoglobin A1C levels, and comprehensive metabolic profile. Angela decided to try metformin, inexpensive and taken orally. It's best to add metformin slowly, starting with one tablet before bed for one week and then increasing to one a.m. and p.m. and sometimes even two a.m. and two p.m.

I was optimistic for Angela. Her fasting insulin level was too high even though she was dedicated to her exercise and diet. Perhaps, her fatigue and her history of erratic periods being part of the same problem. Based on hormone levels, we started her on natural progesterone before bed as well as a low-dose biological thyroid.

Three weeks later, I emailed her and received this response:

> Hi Doctor Birken!
>
> I can see a difference already. I've lost weight. Only 5 pounds, but have more energy. And my last period was lighter.
>
> I'm excited!
> Thanks.

Good news, I thought. But time will tell. At three months, my office called her as a reminder to recheck her fasting insulin/hemoglobin A1C, comprehensive metabolic profile, thyroid, and progesterone. Angela came in for the review.

Immediately, I saw the difference. Not only had she lost weight but her skin looked healthier. Her cheerful personality was back. And best of all, her insulin level was down to twelve and hemoglobin A1C at 5.4—dramatic changes in three months. Thyroid and progesterone levels were optimal as well.

"I feel wonderful," she said enthusiastically. "More energy, better sleep, even my workouts are better. And you know, my periods have remained lighter."

I was delighted to hear this and even more grateful for Dr. Rouzier's tutelage regarding IR patients. "Great, Angela. I'm delighted with your clinical response and repeat labs. The metformin is working well."

She did have some mild diarrhea the first two weeks, but it resolved. This was the perfect choice for her. And she continued to lose weight until she reached her goal. At that time, we considered stopping the metformin, but Angela wanted to continue with just one before bed, a sensible decision.

"Why take the chance on gaining my weight back or even increasing my risk for type II diabetes," she said.

And I agreed.

However, Angela's hormone journey was not over. Three years later, she returned with classic menopausal symptoms: hot flashes, night sweats, lowered libido, and vaginal dryness. Labs confirmed the clinical presentation. Angela was ready to start bio-identical hormones.

"I'm not going to go backward at this point," she said emphatically. "I want to continue to feel vibrant and healthy."

We started her on bio-identical estrogen and testosterone and increased her progesterone dose now that she was menopausal, a way to protect the breasts, bones, and uterus. Angela continued to do well—good energy, sleep, muscle tone, mood, and libido. But three years after becoming menopausal, I saw her for our six-month lab review.

"Your numbers look good Angela. I'm assuming you're feeling well?" I asked not expecting any negative comment. But I did notice a ten-pound weight gain with her vital signs.

"Dr. Birken, I do feel well. But I've gained weight again. Over the past four months. Don't know why." Her smile faded. "I know the metformin is keeping my fasting insulin level steady, and my hemoglobin A1C is the lowest it's ever been." She paused. "What's going on?" she asked with exasperation.

It was true. Angela's labs values, estrogen, progesterone, testosterone, thyroid, DHEA, and thyroid were in the perfect optimal range. And she was correct about her fasting insulin and hemoglobin A1C levels, both low on just one metformin 500 mg tablet before bed.

"Have you changed your exercise program? How about your diet?"

"No!" she said emphatically. "If anything, my diet is cleaner and I exercise more."

I nodded. "Okay, Angela. It's not your insulin resistance." I paused before continuing. Angela's stare widened. "Everyone's physiology is different. For you, the insulin resistance was a problem. But now, there seems to be a problem with your metabolism. I have a suggestion."

Angela leaned forward. "Like what?"

I began to explain the benefits of the many weight-management medications, drugs that can improve metabolism by altering the link between the central nervous system and fat breakdown. For many years, physicians would avoid prescribing these medications for various concerns—overstimulation, possibly increasing blood pressure, sleep disturbances, and even possible addiction. But these medications, used judiciously and under supervision, are actually safe, well-tolerated, and most importantly, extremely effective. The trick is to find the one that works and without side effects. Interestingly, the FDA recommends using the drugs under certain conditions: a body mass index of thirty or higher, or twenty-seven or higher with other associated conditions such as elevated blood pressure and diabetes. And they recommend only for three months, a condition imposed on the pharmaceutical companies to prevent them from erroneous advertising/promotional approaches. Under a physician's supervision and for some individuals, continuous use of one or both of these medications is safe and effective for preventing weight gain. From the *European Association for the Study of Obesity*:

> Obesity management leads to marked improvements in blood glucose control, hypertension, dyslipidemia, and other co-morbidities like osteoarthritis as well as to a reduction in the risk (and severity) of obstructive sleep apnea. As excessive weight plays also an important role in the development of cancer, gout and depression, treatment of obesity could be beneficial or at least preventive in their further deterioration. Successful weight loss has also been shown to improve quality of life, mobility, daily function, and psychological well-being; pharmacotherapy may potentiate these effects. Many of these drugs are purported to operate by strengthening endogenous energy regulation systems and moderating appetite sensations. These have the potential to help the obese gain better control over their eating behavior, and limit their energy intake, making weight management easier.

I have taken many hours of continuing education credit courses from the *American Obesity Association*, studied the indications, side effects, and effectiveness of all weight-management medications, as well as the combination use of these drugs. For Angela, although not obese, I recommend a low-dose, short-term use of a medication called phentermine, an inexpensive sympathomimetic drug. While there can be side effects, such as overstimulation and insomnia, it is usually well tolerated and effective. For those patients who do not tolerate phentermine, or have no clinical response, we try other medications to reduce weight. Of course, diet, exercise, nutritional, and psychological training and education is necessary. But, for Angela, I knew her eating habits were good.

Angela took a low-dose phentermine for three months with great success, losing twelve pounds, and with no side effects. However, if she ever faced the same weight dilemma in the future, I would consider another three months use of a diet pill.

"Thanks, Dr. Birken," she said during one of her follow-up hormone reviews. "I can't tell you how well I feel on the hormones and especially with my weight. What a difference this has made on my overall vitality and even my emotions."

Today, Angela maintains a normal body weight while on her BHRT protocol and a single dose of metformin before bed. Her blood chemistries, including her fasting insulin and hemoglobin A1C levels, remain normal as well as her annual mammograms and bone density testing every three years. While usually pleased with our insulin resistant treatments, I still regret not being aware of its prevalence and treatment options in the past. A common hormone problem, but sadly, often missed.

7

Hormone Optimization: A Work in Progress

The good physician treats the disease; the great physician treats the patient who has the disease.

Sir William Osler

Hopefully, these presented clinical vignettes—composites of actual patients—have been an informative method not only to educate and enlighten but also to reveal the complexities of the art of medicine. While knowledge and skill are essential for proper medical care, understanding the patient's needs and concerns, the ability to assimilate dialogue with facts, to communicate effectively, and to formulate a plan, both simply and economically, are the physician's goal. And yet, today, due to the draconian constraints imposed by managed

health care, the fear of medical liability, and pharmaceutical companies' persistent and pervasive influences,
physicians are restricted in adapting the "father of mod-
ern medicine," Dr. William Osler's doctrine, considered a
tenet that speaks to treating the patient holistically rather
than as with a single disease.

My traditional medical training—thorough, demand-
ing, and comprehensive—approaches each problem as
a separate entity, with emphasis on medications and
surgeries as treatment options. While a necessary part
of health care, the views can be restrictive. I believe in
the benefits of other related disciplines such as nutrition, naturopathy, and the myriad "Eastern" medicine's concepts, and yet Western medicine continues
to purport its approaches. And while it is necessary to
promote scientific research, there are evidence-based
studies that are practically and highly therapeutic.

> *Natural forces within us are the true healers
> of disease.*
>
> —HIPPOCRATES

My criticisms are not meant to malign the "miracles" of
medications, the development of antibiotics to fight the
multitude of infectious disease, the chemotherapeutic
advances for cancer, and the evolution of mental health
drugs, so necessary for those unfortunately inflicted,

but to appeal to health care providers to look beyond what we are taught, and to seek alternatives to conventional protocols. Sadly, despite all the new scientific discoveries and research, the quality of life continues to deteriorate. Again, from Dr. Donovitz:

> For all its advances, medicine seems to not work for us. Death still claims us. In the United States, the leading causes of death are heart disease, cancer, lower respiratory disease, and stroke (cerebrovascular diseases). Many of us die from accidents, and then the next most common causes of death are Alzheimer's disease, influenza and pneumonia and a trio know as nephritis, nephrotic syndrome, and nephrosis, or kidney disease. We are becoming increasing overweight; over one-third of Americans are obese, and another one-third are overweight. These rates are more than doubled since the nineteen-seventies.

How do bio-identical hormones apply to this crisis? As discussed within these stories, "natural" hormones can change lives by increasing energy, improving sleep, reducing aches and pains, stabilizing mood, increasing metabolism and mental clarity, enhancing libido, and heightening a sense of well-being. Do all patients have these responses? No. Do some see no improvement? Infrequently, but yes. But the majority do experience a stronger and more youthful vitality. And, as research suggests, a lower risk for aged-related diseases. The science is readily available for clinicians, if they can transcend the pharmaceutical companies' influence. Again, Dr. Neal Rouzier from his book:

> The most deceptive information we hear is "aging is normal." The decline (cognitive, physical, emotional) we experience is "normal" and we should just learn to live with it. We should fall prey to osteoporosis, heart disease, Alzheimer's, or cancer—no one lives forever. More importantly, some say, no one can prevent or improve this decline. As a doctor and a patient, this kind of apathy is frustrating. I'm excited to say that there is a silver lining. As I delved into the genre of this new research I found that major esteemed medical institutions felt the same way and were researching hormones for their role in health and well-being. Hormones, it appeared, were the key to a longer, heathier life.

Life progresses and changes—a natural flow to our existence. And yet, there is a medically sound approach to enhance the quality of life. While continuing to emphasize healthy eating, regular exercise, and mindful meditation, the clinician must also look beyond traditional medical concepts.

Again, from Sir William Osler's teachings to medical students:

> The practice of medicine is an art, not a trade; a calling, not a business; a calling in which your heart will be exercised equally with your head. Often the best part of your work will have nothing to do with potions and powders, but with the exercise of an influence of the strong upon the weak, of the righteous upon the wicked, of the wise upon the foolish.

With optimism and enthusiasm, I look forward to learning new studies and concepts in natural, bio-identical hormone advances. And more importantly, as a physician, to educate and advise my patients for their well-being, and especially, long-lasting health.

About the Author

After receiving his medical degree from *Boston University School of Medicine* in 1976, Dr. Randy Birken completed his residency at *Baylor College of Medicine* in 1980 after serving as chief resident, eventually devoting his practice to female pelvic reconstruction surgery and uro-gynecology with medical offices in Texas and Colorado.

He added bio-identical hormone optimization to his medical services after training with Dr. Neal Rouzier, and later with Dr. Gary Donovitz, incorporating *BioTe* pellet therapy for both men and women. Also, he completed post graduate training with the *Cenegenics Education and Research Foundation.*

In 2000, Dr. Birken completed his master's degree in liberal arts and taught college literature to undergraduates as well as a lecturer for a series on "Medicine and Literature" presented to medical students. He has authored several scientific papers as well as two collections of short stories, a novel, and a non-fiction book.

Dr. Birken is a volunteer physician at the Interfaith Clinic for indigent patients and has attended three medical missionary trips to Guatemala.

He has served as Clinical Assistant Professor at *Baylor College of Medicine* and is on the medical advisory board with *BioTE Medical.*

Dr. Birken embraces healthy living with regular fitness and proper diet. He and his wife, Liz, live in The Woodlands, Texas and Steamboat Springs, Colorado.

91716788R00059

Made in the USA
Lexington, KY
25 June 2018